OSTEOPOROSIS DIET COOKBOOK FOR WOMEN

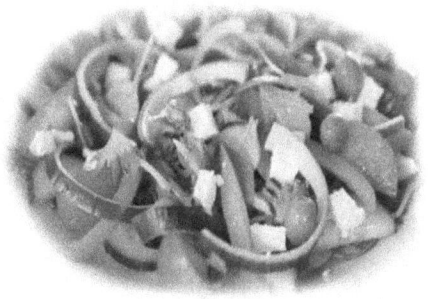

The Ultimate Dietary Guide for Women with Osteoporosis: Rich in Calcium and Bone Health

DR.LINDA MCDANIEL

INTRODUCTION

Welcome to the Osteoporosis Diet Cookbook for Women – a culinary journey designed to empower and enrich the lives of those navigating the challenges of osteoporosis. As a doctor specializing in bone health, I've witnessed firsthand the profound impact that diet can have on managing this condition. Through this cookbook, I aim to provide more than just recipes; I offer a comprehensive guide brimming with nutritious and flavorful dishes specifically crafted to combat inflammation and enhance bone health.

Osteoporosis isn't just a condition; it's a journey, one that demands attention to every aspect of life, including the food we eat. But eating for bone health doesn't have to be bland or restrictive. In fact, it can be a celebration of flavor, texture, and nourishment. Within these pages, you'll discover a treasure trove of recipes carefully curated to tantalize your taste buds while supporting your body's natural defenses against osteoporosis.

From hearty breakfasts to satisfying dinners, each recipe is thoughtfully crafted with ingredients rich in vitamins, minerals, and anti-inflammatory properties essential for bone health. But this cookbook is more than just a collection of recipes – it's a roadmap to a healthier, more vibrant life. Alongside each dish, you'll find invaluable tips and insights into the science behind bone health, empowering you to make informed choices that resonate with your unique dietary needs.

Whether you're newly diagnosed or a seasoned warrior in the battle against osteoporosis, this cookbook is your companion on the path to better bone health. So, join me as we embark on a culinary adventure, one filled with delicious flavors, nourishing ingredients, and the promise of stronger, healthier bones. Let's cook our way to vitality and wellness together.

Here's to your health, happiness, and a future filled with strong, resilient bones.

With warm regards, Dr. Linda McDaniel

TABLE OF CONTENT

INTRODUCTION _____ 3

CHAPTER 1: _____ 7

Understanding Osteoporosis _____ 7

Types of Osteoporosis: _____ 7

Causes of Osteoporosis: _____ 7

Symptoms of Osteoporosis: _____ 8

Prevention of Osteoporosis: _____ 8

CHAPTER 2: _____ 11

Maintaining a healthy diet _____ 11

CHAPTER 3: _____ 15

Dietary Plan to follow _____ 15

CHAPTER 4: _____ 19

Breakfast: _____ 19

Dinner: _____ 34

Dessert: _____ 41

Snacks: _____ 51

CONCLUSION_____ 61

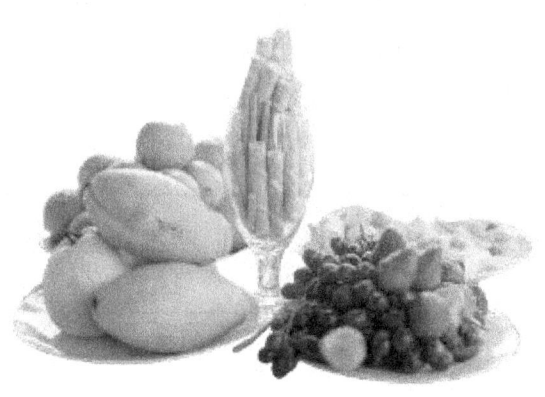

CHAPTER 1:

Understanding Osteoporosis

Osteoporosis is a common bone condition that weakens bones, making them more prone to fractures. In this essay, we'll discuss the different types of osteoporosis, what causes it, its symptoms, and how to prevent it.

Types of Osteoporosis:

Primary Osteoporosis: Linked to aging and hormonal changes, affecting mainly older adults and postmenopausal women.

Secondary Osteoporosis: Caused by other health conditions or medications.

Idiopathic Juvenile Osteoporosis: Rare in children, with no clear cause.

Causes of Osteoporosis:

Hormonal Changes: Decreased estrogen in women and testosterone in men.

Poor Nutrition: Not getting enough calcium, vitamin D, or other vital nutrients.

Lifestyle Factors: Lack of exercise, smoking, excessive alcohol, and poor diet.

Medical Conditions: Rheumatoid arthritis, thyroid problems, and others.

Medications: Long-term use of corticosteroids or certain cancer treatments.

Symptoms of Osteoporosis:

Often no symptoms until a fracture occurs.

Back pain from vertebral fractures.

Loss of height and stooped posture.

Fractures with minimal trauma.

Prevention of Osteoporosis:

- Eat a balanced diet rich in calcium, vitamin D, and protein.
- Exercise regularly, focusing on weight-bearing and balance exercises.
- Avoid smoking, limit alcohol, and maintain a healthy weight.
- Get bone density screenings as recommended by your doctor.

- Consider medications if at high risk for fractures.
- Prevent falls by removing hazards at home and improving balance.

Osteoporosis is a serious condition, but it can be managed and prevented with the right knowledge and lifestyle choices. By understanding its types, causes, symptoms, and preventive measures, individuals can take proactive steps to protect their bone health and enjoy a better quality of life.

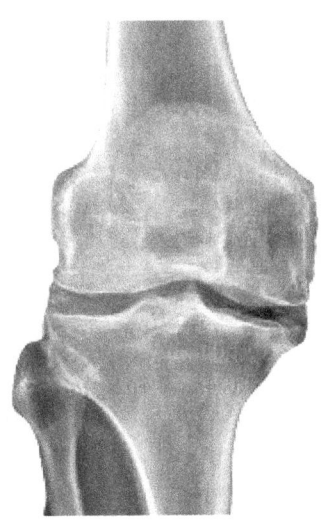

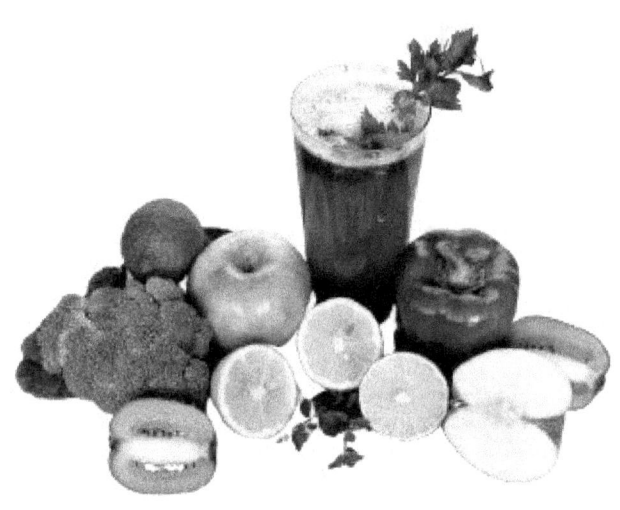

CHAPTER 2:

Maintaining a healthy diet

Maintaining a healthy diet is essential for women with osteoporosis to support bone health and overall well-being. Here's a concise guide on foods to eat and avoid for an osteoporosis diet:

- ➢ **Foods to Eat:**
    - o Calcium-Rich Foods: Calcium is crucial for bone strength. Include dairy items in your diet, such as cheese, yogurt, and milk. Non-dairy sources include leafy greens (kale, broccoli), fortified cereals, and canned fish with bones (sardines, salmon).
    - o Vitamin D Sources: Vitamin D aids calcium absorption. Include fortified foods (milk, orange juice, cereals) and fatty fish (salmon, tuna) in your diet. The body produces vitamin D with the aid of sun exposure.
    - o Protein: Protein is essential for bone formation. Choose lean meats, poultry, fish, eggs, beans, nuts, and seeds to meet your protein needs.

- Magnesium-Rich Foods: Magnesium supports bone health and metabolism. Consume magnesium-rich foods like nuts, seeds, whole grains, legumes, and leafy greens.
- Vitamin K: Vitamin K plays a role in bone mineralization. Incorporate foods such as spinach, kale, broccoli, Brussels sprouts, and green beans into your meals.
- Fruits and Vegetables: Colorful fruits and vegetables provide antioxidants and other nutrients beneficial for overall health. Aim for a variety of fruits and vegetables daily to support bone health and reduce inflammation.
- Healthy Fats: Omega-3 fatty acids found in fish, flaxseeds, and walnuts have anti-inflammatory properties and may support bone health.

➢ **Foods to Limit or Avoid:**

- High-Sodium Foods: Excessive sodium intake can increase calcium excretion and weaken bones. Limit processed foods, canned soups, salty snacks, and fast food.

o Caffeine and Alcohol: High caffeine and alcohol consumption can interfere with calcium absorption and increase bone loss. Limit coffee, tea, soda, and alcoholic beverages.

o Excess Animal Protein: While protein is essential, too much animal protein may increase calcium excretion. Consume lean meats and balance animal protein with plant-based sources.

o Sugary Foods and Beverages: High sugar intake may interfere with calcium absorption and promote inflammation. Limit sweets, sugary drinks, and processed snacks.

o Excessive Phosphorus: High intake of phosphorus-rich foods like processed meats, sodas, and some convenience foods may disrupt calcium balance. Choose whole foods and balance phosphorus intake with calcium-rich foods.

an osteoporosis diet for women should emphasize calcium-rich foods, vitamin D sources, lean proteins, magnesium-rich foods, vitamin K, fruits, vegetables, and healthy fats. It's also essential to limit sodium, caffeine, alcohol, excess animal protein, sugary foods, sugary drinks, and excessive phosphorus. By following a balanced diet and making smart food choices, women can support bone health, reduce inflammation, and achieve optimum overall health.

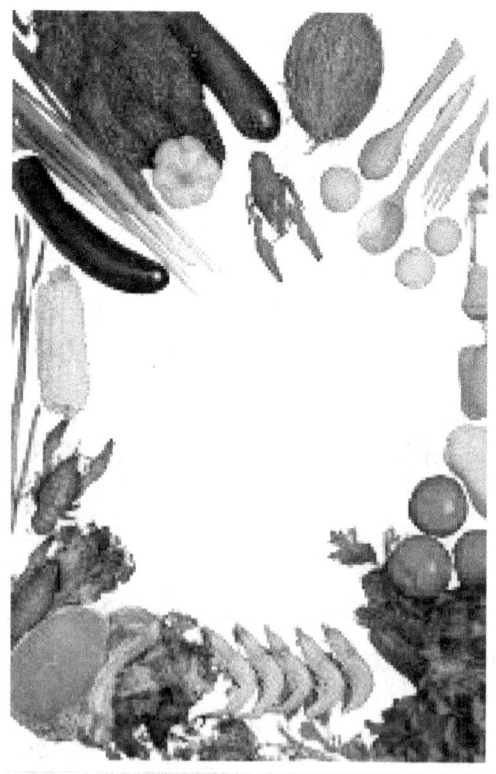

CHAPTER 3:

Dietary Plan to follow

Following an osteoporosis diet for women involves making conscious food choices to support bone health, reduce inflammation, and promote overall well-being. Here's a step-by-step guide on how to follow an osteoporosis diet effectively:

Educate Yourself: Learn about the importance of nutrition in managing osteoporosis. Understand which foods are rich in essential nutrients like calcium, vitamin D, magnesium, and vitamin K, and how they contribute to bone health.

Consult a Healthcare Professional: Before making significant changes to your diet, consult with a healthcare provider or a registered dietitian specializing in bone health. They can provide personalized recommendations based on your medical history, nutritional needs, and specific dietary requirements.

Plan Balanced Meals: Design your meals to include a variety of nutrient-dense foods. Aim for a balanced combination of lean proteins, whole grains, fruits, vegetables, dairy or dairy alternatives, and healthy fats in each meal.

Focus on Calcium-Rich Foods: Incorporate calcium-rich foods into your daily diet to support bone density. Include dairy products like milk, yogurt, and cheese, as well as non-dairy sources such as leafy greens, fortified cereals, tofu, and canned fish with bones.

Include Vitamin D Sources: Ensure adequate intake of vitamin D to enhance calcium absorption and bone mineralization. Incorporate foods fortified with vitamin D, such as milk, orange juice, and cereals, as well as fatty fish like salmon, tuna, and mackerel. Additionally, spend time outdoors to allow your skin to produce vitamin D from sunlight.

Opt for Lean Proteins: Choose lean protein sources like poultry, fish, beans, lentils, nuts, and seeds to support muscle strength and overall health. Limit red meat and processed meats, which may contribute to inflammation and negatively impact bone health when consumed in excess.

Prioritize Magnesium and Vitamin K: Include foods rich in magnesium and vitamin K to support bone metabolism and calcium utilization.

Consume magnesium-rich foods like nuts, seeds, whole grains, legumes, and leafy greens, and incorporate vitamin K sources such as spinach, kale, broccoli, Brussels sprouts, and green beans into your meals.

Limit Inflammatory Foods: Reduce your intake of foods that promote inflammation, such as processed foods, sugary snacks, refined grains, and foods high in saturated and trans fats. Instead, focus on whole, unprocessed foods that provide essential nutrients and antioxidants to support bone health.

Monitor Sodium and Caffeine Intake: Limit your consumption of high-sodium foods, as excess sodium can increase calcium excretion and weaken bones. Be mindful of your caffeine intake, as excessive caffeine consumption may interfere with calcium absorption and contribute to bone loss.

Stay Hydrated: Keep Yourself Hydrated: To promote general health and hydration, sip lots of water throughout the day. Limit sugary beverages and opt for water, herbal teas, and unsweetened beverages to minimize calorie intake and reduce the risk of dehydration.

Practice Portion Control: Pay attention to portion sizes to maintain a healthy weight and prevent overeating. Opt for smaller, more frequent meals and snacks to help regulate blood sugar levels and energy levels throughout the day.

Be Consistent: Make sustainable dietary changes and incorporate healthy eating habits into your lifestyle. Consistency is key to long-term success in managing osteoporosis and promoting overall health and well-being.

By following these guidelines and making informed food choices, women can effectively follow an osteoporosis diet that supports bone health, reduces inflammation, and enhances overall quality of life.

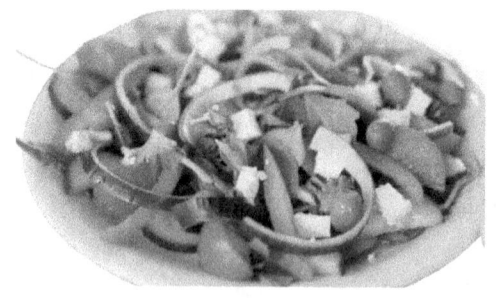

CHAPTER 4:

Breakfast:

➤ Yogurt Parfait

Ingredients:

- 1/2 cup low-fat Greek yogurt

- 1/4 cup granola (low-sugar)

- 1/2 cup mixed berries (strawberries, blueberries, raspberries)

- 1 tablespoon honey or maple syrup (optional)
Preparation:

1. In a serving glass or bowl, layer Greek yogurt, granola, and mixed berries.

2. Drizzle with honey or maple syrup if desired.

3. Serve immediately.

Cooking Time: 5 minutes

Nutritional Value (per serving): Calories: 250, Protein: 12g, Calcium: 150mg, Vitamin D: 0 IU

➤ Spinach and Feta Omelette

Ingredients: 2 eggs, 1/2 cup fresh spinach leaves, 1/4 cup crumbled feta cheese, Salt and pepper to taste, 1 teaspoon olive oil

Preparation:

1. In a bowl, beat the eggs and season with salt and pepper.

2. Heat olive oil in a non-stick skillet over medium heat.

3. Add spinach to the skillet and cook until wilted.

4. Pour beaten eggs over the spinach and cook until set.

5. Sprinkle feta cheese over one half of the omelette and fold the other half over the filling.

6. Cook for another minute until the cheese melts.

7. Serve hot.

Cooking Time: 10 minutes

Nutritional Value (per serving): Calories: 280, Protein: 20g, Calcium: 200mg, Vitamin D: 60 IU

➢ Overnight Oats

Ingredients: 1/2 cup rolled oats, 1/2 cup low-fat milk or almond milk, 1/4 cup Greek yogurt, 1 tablespoon chia seeds, 1/2 teaspoon vanilla extract, 1 tablespoon honey or maple syrup (optional), 1/4 cup sliced almonds or mixed nuts, 1/2 cup diced fruits (apple, banana, berries)

Preparation:

1. In a jar or container, combine rolled oats, milk, Greek yogurt, chia seeds, vanilla extract, and honey or maple syrup (if using).

2. Stir well to combine all ingredients.

3. Cover and refrigerate overnight.

4. In the morning, stir the oats mixture and top with sliced almonds or mixed nuts and diced fruits.

5. Serve chilled.

Cooking Time: 5 minutes (plus overnight refrigeration)

Nutritional Value (per serving): Calories: 350, Protein: 15g, Calcium: 200mg,

Vitamin D: 0 IU

➢ Avocado Toast

Ingredients:

- 1 slice whole grain bread, toasted, 1/2 ripe avocado, mashed, 1 teaspoon lemon juice, Pinch of salt and pepper, Optional toppings: sliced tomato, sprouts, poached egg

Preparation:

1. Toast the whole grain bread until golden brown.

2. In a small bowl, mash the ripe avocado with lemon juice, salt, and pepper.

3. Spread the mashed avocado evenly onto the toasted bread.

4. Top with sliced tomato, sprouts, or a poached egg if desired.

5. Serve immediately.

Cooking Time: 5 minutes

Nutritional Value (per serving): Calories: 200

Protein: 5g, Calcium: 20mg, Vitamin D: 0 IU

➤ Berry Smoothie Bowl

Ingredients:

- 1/2 cup frozen mixed berries, 1/2 ripe banana, 1/2 cup low-fat Greek yogurt, 1/4 cup low-fat milk or almond milk, 1 tablespoon chia seeds, Toppings: sliced almonds, shredded coconut, fresh berries, granola

Preparation:

1. In a blender, combine frozen berries, banana, Greek yogurt, milk, and chia seeds.

2. Blend until smooth and creamy.

3. Pour the smoothie into a bowl.

4. Top with sliced almonds, shredded coconut, fresh berries, and granola.

5. Serve immediately with a spoon.

Cooking Time: 5 minutes

Nutritional Value (per serving): Calories: 250, Protein: 12g, Calcium: 150mg

Vitamin D: 0 IU

➤ Veggie Breakfast Burrito

Ingredients: 1 whole wheat tortilla, 1 egg, scrambled, 1/4 cup black beans, rinsed and drained, 2 tablespoons diced bell peppers, 2 tablespoons diced tomatoes, 2 tablespoons chopped spinach, 2 tablespoons shredded low-fat cheese, Salsa or avocado for serving (optional)

Preparation:

1. Heat a non-stick skillet over medium heat.

2. Add scrambled eggs, black beans, bell peppers, tomatoes, and spinach to the skillet.

3. Cook until eggs are scrambled and vegetables are tender.

4. Warm the whole wheat tortilla in the skillet or microwave.

5. Spoon the egg and vegetable mixture onto the tortilla and sprinkle with shredded cheese.

6. Roll up the tortilla to form a burrito.

7. Serve with salsa or avocado if desired.

Cooking Time: 10 minutes

Nutritional Value (per serving): Calories: 300, Protein: 15g, Calcium: 100mg, Vitamin D: 40 IU

Lunch:

➢ Grilled Salmon Salad

Ingredients: 4 oz salmon fillet, 2 cups mixed greens, 1/2 cup cherry tomatoes, halved, 1/4 cucumber, sliced, 1/4 avocado, sliced, 1 tablespoon olive oil, 1 tablespoon balsamic vinegar, Salt and pepper to taste

Preparation:

1. Season salmon fillet with salt and pepper.

2. Grill salmon over medium-high heat for 4-5 minutes per side or until cooked through.

3. In a large bowl, toss mixed greens, cherry tomatoes, cucumber, and avocado with olive oil and balsamic vinegar.

4. Top salad with grilled salmon.

5. Serve immediately.

Cooking Time: 10 minutes

Nutritional Value (per serving): Calories: 350 Protein: 25g Calcium: 50mg

Vitamin D: 120 IU

➤ Quinoa and Vegetable Stir-Fry

Ingredients: 1/2 cup quinoa 1 cup water or low-sodium vegetable broth, 1 tablespoon olive oil, 1/2 onion, diced, 1 bell pepper, sliced, 1 cup broccoli florets, 1 carrot, julienned, 2 cloves garlic, minced, 2 tablespoons low-sodium soy sauce, 1 tablespoon rice vinegar, 1 teaspoon sesame oil, Sesame seeds for garnish

Preparation:

1. Rinse quinoa under cold water. In a saucepan, bring water or vegetable broth to a boil. Add quinoa, reduce heat, cover, and simmer for 15 minutes or until water is absorbed.

2. In a large skillet or wok, heat olive oil over medium-high heat. Add onion, bell pepper, broccoli, carrot, and garlic. Stir-fry for 5-6 minutes until vegetables are tender-crisp.

3. Stir in cooked quinoa, soy sauce, rice vinegar, and sesame oil. Cook for an additional 2-3 minutes, stirring occasionally.

4. Garnish with sesame seeds before serving.

Cooking Time: 25 minutes

Nutritional Value (per serving): Calories: 300, Protein: 10g. Calcium: 60mg, Vitamin D: 0 IU

➤ Turkey and Vegetable Wrap

Ingredients: 1 whole wheat tortilla, 3 oz sliced turkey breast, 1/4 avocado, mashed, 1/4 cup shredded lettuce, 1/4 cup sliced cucumber, 1/4 cup shredded carrots, 1 tablespoon hummus, Salt and pepper to taste

Preparation:

1. Lay the whole wheat tortilla on a flat surface.

2. Spread mashed avocado and hummus evenly over the tortilla.

3. Layer sliced turkey breast, shredded lettuce, cucumber, and shredded carrots on top.

4. Season with salt and pepper to taste.

5. Roll up the tortilla tightly to form a wrap.

6. Cut the wrap in half diagonally before serving.
   Cooking Time: 5 minutes

Nutritional Value (per serving):

Calories: 250, Protein: 20g, Calcium: 40mg

Vitamin D: 0 IU

➤ Lentil and Vegetable Soup

Ingredients: 1/2 cup dried lentils, rinsed, 4 cups low-sodium vegetable broth, 1 tablespoon olive oil, 1/2 onion, diced, 2 carrots, diced, 2 celery stalks, diced, 2 cloves garlic, minced, 1 teaspoon ground cumin, 1/2 teaspoon smoked paprika, Salt and pepper to taste, Fresh parsley for garnish

Preparation:

1. In a large pot, heat olive oil over medium heat. Add diced onion, carrots, celery, and garlic. Cook until vegetables are softened, about 5 minutes.

2. Stir in dried lentils, vegetable broth, ground cumin, and smoked paprika. Bring to a boil, then reduce heat and simmer for 20-25 minutes or until lentils are tender.

3. Season with salt and pepper to taste.

4. Ladle soup into bowls and garnish with fresh parsley before serving.

Cooking Time: 30 minutes

Nutritional Value (per serving): Calories: 200, Protein: 12g, Calcium: 60mg

Vitamin D: 0 IU

> ## Tuna Salad Stuffed Avocado

Ingredients: 1 ripe avocado, halved and pitted, 1 can (5 oz) tuna in water, drained, 1 tablespoon Greek yogurt, 1 teaspoon lemon juice, 1/4 cup diced cucumber, 1/4 cup diced tomatoes, 1 tablespoon chopped fresh parsley, Salt and pepper to taste

Preparation:

1. In a bowl, mix together drained tuna, Greek yogurt, lemon juice, diced cucumber, diced tomatoes, and chopped fresh parsley.

2. Season with salt and pepper to taste.

3. Spoon the tuna salad mixture into the halved avocado.

4. Serve immediately.

Cooking Time: 10 minutes

Nutritional Value (per serving): Calories: 250, Protein: 20g

Calcium: 40mg

Vitamin D: 0 IU

➤ Veggie and Hummus Wrap

Ingredients: 1 whole wheat tortilla, 2 tablespoons hummus, 1/4 cup shredded lettuce, 1/4 cup sliced cucumber, 1/4 cup shredded carrots, 1/4 cup sliced bell peppers, Salt and pepper to taste

Preparation:

1. Lay the whole wheat tortilla on a flat surface.

2. Spread hummus evenly over the tortilla.

3. Layer shredded lettuce, sliced cucumber, shredded carrots, and sliced bell peppers on top of the hummus.

4. Season with salt and pepper to taste.

5. Roll up the tortilla tightly to form a wrap.

6. Cut the wrap in half diagonally before serving.

Cooking Time: 5 minutes

Nutritional Value (per serving):

Calories: 200

Protein: 6g

Calcium: 30mg

Vitamin D: 0 IU

➤ Egg Salad Stuffed Tomatoes

Ingredients: 2 large tomatoes, 2 hard-boiled eggs, chopped, 2 tablespoons Greek yogurt, 1 teaspoon Dijon mustard, 1 tablespoon chopped chives, Salt and pepper to taste

Preparation:

1. Cut the tops off the tomatoes and scoop out the seeds and pulp to create a hollow space.

2. In a bowl, mix together chopped hard-boiled eggs, Greek yogurt, Dijon mustard, chopped chives, salt, and pepper.

3. Spoon the egg salad mixture into the hollowed-out tomatoes.

4. Serve immediately.

Cooking Time: 15 minutes

Nutritional Value (per serving): Calories: 150

Protein: 10g

Calcium: 60mg

Vitamin D: 0 IU

> ## Chickpea and Vegetable Salad

Ingredients: 1 can (15 oz) chickpeas, rinsed and drained, 1/2 cup diced cucumber, 1/2 cup diced tomatoes, 1/4 cup diced red onion, 1/4 cup chopped parsley 1 tablespoon olive oil, 1 tablespoon lemon juice, Salt and pepper to taste

Preparation:

1. In a large bowl, combine chickpeas, diced cucumber, diced tomatoes, diced red onion, and chopped parsley.

2. Drizzle olive oil and lemon juice over the salad.

3. Season with salt and pepper to taste.

4. Toss until well combined.

5. Serve chilled or at room temperature.

Cooking Time: 10 minutes

Nutritional Value (per serving): Calories: 250

Protein: 10g

Calcium: 50mg

Vitamin D: 0 IU

➤ Caprese Salad

Ingredients: 1 cup cherry tomatoes, halved, 1/2 cup fresh mozzarella balls, 1/4 cup fresh basil leaves, 1 tablespoon balsamic vinegar, 1 tablespoon olive oil, Salt and pepper to taste

Preparation:

1. In a bowl, combine cherry tomatoes, fresh mozzarella balls, and fresh basil leaves.

2. Drizzle balsamic vinegar and olive oil over the salad.

3. Season with salt and pepper to taste.

4. Toss until well combined.

5. Serve immediately.

Cooking Time: 5 minutes

Nutritional Value (per serving):

Calories: 200

Protein: 10g

Calcium: 150mg

Vitamin D: 0 IU

Dinner:

➢ Baked Salmon with Roasted Vegetables

Ingredients: 4 oz salmon fillet, 1 cup mixed vegetables (bell peppers, zucchini, carrots), 1 tablespoon olive oil, Salt and pepper to taste, Fresh lemon wedges for serving

Preparation:

1. Preheat the oven to 400°F (200°C).

2. Place the salmon fillet on a baking sheet lined with parchment paper.

3. Toss the mixed vegetables with olive oil, salt, and pepper, and arrange them around the salmon on the baking sheet.

4. Bake for 15-20 minutes, or until the salmon is cooked through and the vegetables are tender.

5. Serve hot with fresh lemon wedges.

Cooking Time: 20 minutes

Nutritional Value (per serving): Calories: 300, Protein: 25g, Calcium: 50mg

Vitamin D: 150 IU

➤ Chicken and Vegetable Stir-Fry

Ingredients: 4 oz boneless, skinless chicken breast, sliced, 1 cup mixed vegetables (broccoli, bell peppers, snap peas), 1 tablespoon olive oil, 2 tablespoons low-sodium soy sauce, 1 tablespoon hoisin sauce, 1 teaspoon cornstarch, Cooked brown rice for serving

Preparation:

1. In a small bowl, whisk together soy sauce, hoisin sauce, and cornstarch. Set aside.

2. Heat olive oil in a large skillet or wok over medium-high heat. Add sliced chicken breast and cook until browned and cooked through, about 5-6 minutes. Remove chicken from the skillet and set aside.

3. In the same skillet, add mixed vegetables and stir-fry for 4-5 minutes until tender-crisp.

4. Return cooked chicken to the skillet and pour the sauce mixture over the chicken and vegetables. Cook for an additional 2-3 minutes, stirring continuously, until the sauce thickens.

5. Serve stir-fry over cooked brown rice.

Cooking Time: 20 minutes & Nutritional Value (per serving): Calories: 300, Protein: 25g, Calcium: 50mg, Vitamin D: 0 IU

➤ Lentil Soup with Spinach

Ingredients: 1/2 cup dried lentils, rinsed, 4 cups low-sodium vegetable broth, 1 tablespoon olive oil, 1/2 onion, diced, 2 carrots, diced, 2 celery stalks, diced, 2 cloves garlic, minced, 1 teaspoon ground cumin, 1/2 teaspoon smoked paprika, 2 cups fresh spinach leaves, Salt and pepper to taste

Preparation:

1. In a large pot, heat olive oil over medium heat. Add diced onion, carrots, celery, and garlic. Cook until vegetables are softened, about 5 minutes.

2. Stir in dried lentils, vegetable broth, ground cumin, and smoked paprika. Bring to a boil, then reduce heat and simmer for 20-25 minutes or until lentils are tender.

3. Add fresh spinach leaves to the soup and cook for an additional 2-3 minutes until wilted.

4. Season with salt and pepper to taste and Serve hot.

Cooking Time: 30 minutes

Nutritional Value (per serving): Calories: 200, Protein: 12g, Calcium: 60mg, Vitamin D: 0 IU

➤ Baked Chicken and Sweet Potato Wedges

Ingredients: 4 oz chicken breast, boneless and skinless, 1 medium sweet potato, cut into wedges, 1 tablespoon olive oil, 1 teaspoon paprika, 1/2 teaspoon garlic powder, 1/2 teaspoon onion powder, Salt and pepper to taste, Fresh parsley for garnish

Preparation:

1. Preheat the oven to 400°F (200°C) in a bowl, toss sweet potato wedges with olive oil, paprika, garlic powder, onion powder, salt, and pepper.

2. Place the seasoned sweet potato wedges on a baking sheet lined with parchment paper.

3. Season chicken breast with salt and pepper, and place it on the same baking sheet.

4. Bake for 20-25 minutes, or until the chicken is cooked through and the sweet potato wedges are golden and tender.

5. Garnish with fresh parsley before serving and serve hot.

Cooking Time: 30 minutes & Nutritional Value (per serving): Calories: 300 Protein: 25g, Calcium: 40mg, Vitamin D: 0 IU

➤ Vegetable and Bean Chili

Ingredients: 1 can (15 oz) mixed beans, rinsed and drained, 1 can (14 oz) diced tomatoes, 1 cup low-sodium vegetable broth, 1/2 onion, diced, 1 bell pepper, diced, 1 cup diced zucchini, 2 cloves garlic, minced, 1 tablespoon olive oil, 1 tablespoon chili powder, 1 teaspoon ground cumin, Salt and pepper to taste, Fresh cilantro for garnish

Preparation:

1. Heat olive oil in a large pot over medium heat. Add diced onion, bell pepper, zucchini, and garlic. Cook until vegetables are softened, about 5 minutes.

2. Stir in chili powder and ground cumin, and cook for another minute.

3. Add mixed beans, diced tomatoes, and vegetable broth to the pot. Bring to a boil, then reduce heat and simmer for 20-25 minutes.

4. Season with salt and pepper to taste.

5. Garnish with fresh cilantro before serving then serve hot.

Cooking Time: 30 minutes & Nutritional Value (per serving): Calories: 250, Protein: 10g, Calcium: 50mg, Vitamin D: 0 IU

➤ Baked Cod with Lemon Herb Sauce

Ingredients: 4 oz cod fillet, 1 tablespoon olive oil, 1 tablespoon lemon juice, 1 teaspoon minced garlic, 1 tablespoon chopped fresh parsley, Salt and pepper to taste, Lemon slices for garnish

Preparation:

1. Preheat the oven to 400°F (200°C).

2. In a small bowl, mix together olive oil, lemon juice, minced garlic, chopped fresh parsley, salt, and pepper.

3. Place the cod fillet on a baking sheet lined with parchment paper.

4. Brush the lemon herb sauce over the cod fillet.

5. Bake for 15-20 minutes, or until the cod is opaque and flakes easily with a fork.

6. Garnish with lemon slices before serving and serve hot.

Cooking Time: 20 minutes

Nutritional Value (per serving): Calories: 200 Protein: 20g, Calcium: 40mg, Vitamin D: 0 IU

➤ Veggie and Tofu Stir-Fry

Ingredients: 4 oz firm tofu, cubed, 1 cup mixed vegetables (broccoli, bell peppers, snow peas), 1 tablespoon olive oil, 2 tablespoons low-sodium soy sauce, 1 tablespoon hoisin sauce, 1 teaspoon cornstarch, Cooked brown rice for serving

Preparation:

1. In a small bowl, whisk together soy sauce, hoisin sauce, and cornstarch. Set aside.

2. Heat olive oil in a large skillet or wok over medium-high heat. Add cubed tofu and stir-fry for 4-5 minutes until golden brown.

3. Remove tofu from the skillet and set aside.

4. In the same skillet, add mixed vegetables and stir-fry for 4-5 minutes until tender-crisp.

5. Return cooked tofu to the skillet and pour the sauce mixture over the tofu and vegetables. Cook for an additional 2-3 minutes, stirring continuously, until the sauce thickens.

6. Serve stir-fry over cooked brown rice.

Cooking Time: 20 minutes & Nutritional Value (per serving): Calories: 250, Protein: 15g, Calcium: 50mg, Vitamin D: 0 IU

Dessert:

➤ Baked Apples with Cinnamon

Ingredients:

- 4 medium apples

- 2 tablespoons brown sugar, 1 teaspoon ground cinnamon, 1 tablespoon unsalted butter, melted, 1/4 cup chopped walnuts (optional)

Preparation:

1. Preheat the oven to 375°F (190°C).

2. Core the apples and place them in a baking dish.

3. In a small bowl, mix together brown sugar, cinnamon, melted butter, and chopped walnuts.

4. Spoon the mixture into the center of each apple.

5. Bake for 25-30 minutes or until the apples are tender.

6. Serve warm.

Cooking Time: 30 minutes

Nutritional Value (per serving): Calories: 150 Protein: 1g, Calcium: 10mg, Vitamin D: 0 IU

➤ Frozen Yogurt Bark

Ingredients: 1 cup low-fat Greek yogurt, 2 tablespoons honey or maple syrup, 1/4 cup mixed berries (blueberries, strawberries), 2 tablespoons sliced almonds

Preparation:

1. Line a baking sheet with parchment paper.

2. In a bowl, mix Greek yogurt with honey or maple syrup.

3. Spread the yogurt mixture onto the prepared baking sheet.

4. Sprinkle mixed berries and sliced almonds over the yogurt.

5. Freeze for 2-3 hours until firm.

6. Break into pieces before serving.

Cooking Time: 3 hours

Nutritional Value (per serving):

Calories: 120

Protein: 5g, Calcium: 100mg, Vitamin D: 0 IU

➢ Chia Seed Pudding

Ingredients: 1/4 cup chia seeds, 1 cup low-fat milk or almond milk, 1 tablespoon honey or maple syrup, 1/2 teaspoon vanilla extract, 1/4 cup sliced strawberries, 1/4 cup sliced kiwi
Preparation:

1. In a bowl, whisk together chia seeds, milk, honey or maple syrup, and vanilla extract.

2. Let it sit for 10 minutes, then whisk again to prevent clumping.

3. Cover and refrigerate for at least 2 hours or overnight until thickened.

4. Before serving, top with sliced strawberries and kiwi.

Cooking Time: 2 hours 10 minutes

Nutritional Value (per serving): Calories: 150

Protein: 5g

Calcium: 100mg

Vitamin D: 0 IU

➢ Banana Oatmeal Cookies

Ingredients: 2 ripe bananas, mashed, 1 cup rolled oats, 1/4 cup chopped walnuts, 1/4 cup dried cranberries, 1/2 teaspoon cinnamon, 1/4 teaspoon vanilla extract

Preparation:

1. Preheat the oven to 350°F (175°C). Line a baking sheet with parchment paper.

2. In a bowl, combine mashed bananas, rolled oats, chopped walnuts, dried cranberries, cinnamon, and vanilla extract.

3. Drop spoonfuls of the mixture onto the prepared baking sheet.

4. Bake for 15-20 minutes or until golden brown.

5. Let cool before serving.

Cooking Time: 20 minutes

Nutritional Value (per serving): Calories: 120, Protein: 3g

Calcium: 20mg

Vitamin D: 0 IU

➤ Greek Yogurt Cheesecake

Ingredients: 1 cup low-fat Greek yogurt, 1/4 cup honey, 1 tablespoon lemon juice, 1 teaspoon vanilla extract, 1/2 cup graham cracker crumbs, Fresh berries for topping

Preparation:

1. In a bowl, mix together Greek yogurt, honey, lemon juice, and vanilla extract until smooth.

2. Press graham cracker crumbs into the bottom of serving glasses.

3. Pour the yogurt mixture over the crumbs.

4. Refrigerate for at least 2 hours until set.

5. Top with fresh berries before serving.

Cooking Time: 2 hours

Nutritional Value (per serving): Calories: 150

Protein: 5g

Calcium: 100mg

Vitamin D: 0 IU

➤ Chocolate Avocado Mousse

Ingredients: 2 ripe avocados, 1/4 cup cocoa powder, 1/4 cup honey or maple syrup, 1 teaspoon vanilla extract, Pinch of salt

Preparation:

1. In a food processor, blend avocados, cocoa powder, honey or maple syrup, vanilla extract, and salt until smooth.

2. Divide the mixture into serving glasses.

3. Refrigerate for at least 1 hour before serving.

4. Optional: garnish with shaved dark chocolate or fresh berries.

Cooking Time: 1 hour 10 minutes

Nutritional Value (per serving): Calories: 200

Protein: 2g

Calcium: 10mg

Vitamin D: 0 IU

➤ Berry Crisp

Ingredients: 2 cups mixed berries (blueberries, raspberries, blackberries), 1 tablespoon honey or maple syrup, 1/2 cup rolled oats, 1/4 cup almond flour, 2 tablespoons coconut oil, melted, 1/2 teaspoon cinnamon

Preparation:

1. Preheat the oven to 350°F (175°C). Grease a baking dish with coconut oil.

2. In a bowl, toss mixed berries with honey or maple syrup. Transfer to the prepared baking dish.

3. In another bowl, mix rolled oats, almond flour, melted coconut oil, and cinnamon until crumbly.

4. Sprinkle the oat mixture evenly over the berries.

5. Bake for 25-30 minutes or until the topping is golden brown and the berries are bubbling.

6. Let cool slightly before serving.

Cooking Time: 30 minutes

Nutritional Value (per serving): Calories: 180 Protein: 3g, Calcium: 30mg, Vitamin D: 0 IU

➢ Pumpkin Spice Bites

Ingredients: 1/2 cup pumpkin puree, 1/4 cup almond butter, 1/4 cup maple syrup, 1 teaspoon pumpkin pie spice, 1 cup rolled oats, 1/4 cup shredded coconut

Preparation:

1. In a bowl, mix together pumpkin puree, almond butter, maple syrup, and pumpkin pie spice until well combined.

2. Stir in rolled oats and shredded coconut until evenly distributed.

3. Roll the mixture into small balls and place them on a baking sheet lined with parchment paper.

4. Refrigerate for at least 30 minutes before serving.

5. Optional: roll the bites in additional shredded coconut before refrigerating.

Cooking Time: 30 minutes

Nutritional Value (per serving): Calories: 120, Protein: 3g

Calcium: 20mg

Vitamin D: 0 IU

➤ Coconut Chia Pudding

Ingredients: 1/4 cup chia seeds, 1 cup coconut milk, 2 tablespoons honey or maple syrup, 1/4 teaspoon vanilla extract, Toasted coconut flakes for topping

Preparation:

1. In a bowl, whisk together chia seeds, coconut milk, honey or maple syrup, and vanilla extract.

2. Cover and refrigerate for at least 2 hours or overnight until thickened.

3. Stir well before serving and top with toasted coconut flakes.

Cooking Time: 2 hours 10 minutes

Nutritional Value (per serving):

Calories: 180

Protein: 3g

Calcium: 100mg

Vitamin D: 0 IU

➢ Apple Cinnamon Oat Bars

Ingredients: 2 cups rolled oats, 1/4 cup almond flour, 1 teaspoon ground cinnamon, 1/4 cup honey or maple syrup, 1/4 cup unsweetened applesauce, 1/4 cup almond butter, 1/2 cup diced apples

Preparation:

1. Preheat the oven to 350°F (175°C). Grease a baking dish with coconut oil.

2. In a bowl, mix together rolled oats, almond flour, and ground cinnamon.

3. In another bowl, whisk together honey or maple syrup, applesauce, and almond butter until smooth.

4. Combine wet and dry ingredients, then fold in diced apples.

5. Press the mixture into the prepared baking dish.

6. Bake for 20-25 minutes or until golden brown.

7. Let cool before slicing into bars.

Cooking Time: 25 minutes

Nutritional Value (per serving): Calories: 160 Protein: 4g, Calcium: 20mg, Vitamin D: 0 IU

Snacks:

> ## Yogurt and Berry Smoothie

Ingredients:, 1/2 cup low-fat yogurt, 1/2 cup mixed berries (blueberries, strawberries, raspberries), 1/2 banana, 1/4 cup almond milk, 1 tablespoon honey or maple syrup (optional)
Preparation:

1. Blend all ingredients together until smooth.

2. Add more almond milk if needed to reach desired consistency.

3. Pour into a glass and enjoy.

Preparation Time: 5 minutes

Nutritional Value (per serving):

Calories: 150

Protein: 6g

Calcium: 150mg

Vitamin D: 0 IU

➤ Whole Grain Crackers with Hummus

Ingredients:

- 4 whole grain crackers
- 1/4 cup hummus
- 1 carrot, sliced, 1 celery stalk, sliced

Preparation:

1. Spread hummus evenly onto each cracker.
2. Serve with carrot and celery slices.

Preparation Time: 5 minutes

Nutritional Value (per serving):

Calories: 120

Protein: 5g

Calcium: 40mg

Vitamin D: 0 IU

➢ Greek Yogurt with Granola and Fruit

Ingredients:

- 1/2 cup low-fat Greek yogurt

- 1/4 cup granola (low-sugar)

- 1/4 cup mixed berries (blueberries, strawberries)

Preparation:

1. Spoon Greek yogurt into a bowl.

2. Sprinkle granola and mixed berries over the yogurt.

3. Serve immediately.

Preparation Time: 5 minutes

Nutritional Value (per serving): Calories: 180

Protein: 8g

Calcium: 200mg

Vitamin D: 0 IU

> ## Almond Butter and Banana Slices on Whole Wheat Toast

Ingredients:

- 2 slices whole wheat bread, toasted
- 2 tablespoons almond butter
- 1/2 banana, sliced

Preparation:

1. Spread almond butter evenly onto each slice of toast.

2. Arrange banana slices on top.

3. Serve immediately.

Preparation Time: 5 minutes

Nutritional Value (per serving):

Calories: 250

Protein: 8g

Calcium: 60mg

Vitamin D: 0 IU

➤ Cottage Cheese with Pineapple

Ingredients:

- 1/2 cup low-fat cottage cheese
- 1/2 cup diced pineapple

Preparation:

1. Spoon cottage cheese into a bowl.

2. Top with diced pineapple.

3. Serve chilled.

Preparation Time: 5 minutes

Nutritional Value (per serving):

Calories: 150

Protein: 14g

Calcium: 100mg

Vitamin D: 0 IU

➤ Vegetable Sticks with Yogurt Dip

Ingredients:

- 1 carrot, cut into sticks
- 1 cucumber, cut into sticks
- 1 bell pepper, cut into strips
- 1/2 cup low-fat Greek yogurt
- 1 tablespoon chopped fresh herbs (parsley, dill)
- Salt and pepper to taste

Preparation:

1. Arrange vegetable sticks on a plate.
2. In a small bowl, mix Greek yogurt with chopped herbs, salt, and pepper.
3. Serve vegetable sticks with yogurt dip.

Preparation Time: 10 minutes

Nutritional Value (per serving): Calories: 100

Protein: 8g

Calcium: 100mg

Vitamin D: 0 IU

➤ Trail Mix with Nuts and Dried Fruit

Ingredients:

- 1/4 cup mixed nuts (almonds, walnuts, cashews)
- 2 tablespoons dried cranberries
- 2 tablespoons pumpkin seeds
- 2 tablespoons dark chocolate chips

Preparation:

1. Mix all ingredients together in a bowl.
2. Divide into individual portions.
3. Serve as a snack on-the-go.

Preparation Time: 5 minutes

Nutritional Value (per serving):

Calories: 200

Protein: 5g

Calcium: 40mg

Vitamin D: 0 IU

➢ Rice Cake with Avocado and Tomato

Ingredients:

- 1 rice cake
- 1/4 avocado, mashed
- 1 slice tomato
- Pinch of salt and pepper

Preparation:

1. Spread mashed avocado onto the rice cake.
2. Top with a slice of tomato.
3. Season with salt and pepper.
4. Serve immediately.

Preparation Time: 5 minutes

Nutritional Value (per serving): Calories: 100, Protein: 2g

Calcium: 10mg

Vitamin D: 0 IU

➢ Apple Slices with Peanut Butter

Ingredients:

- 1 apple, sliced
- 2 tablespoons peanut butter

Preparation:

1. Spread peanut butter onto apple slices.
2. Serve immediately.

Preparation Time: 5 minutes

Nutritional Value (per serving):

Calories: 200

Protein: 5g

Calcium: 20mg

Vitamin D: 0 IU

Greek Yogurt with Sliced Almonds and Honey

Ingredients:

- 1/2 cup low-fat Greek yogurt
- 1 tablespoon sliced almonds
- 1 teaspoon honey Preparation:

1. Spoon Greek yogurt into a bowl.

2. Top with sliced almonds and drizzle with honey.

3. Serve immediately.

Preparation Time: 5 minutes

Nutritional Value (per serving):

- Calories: 150
- Protein: 10g
- Calcium: 100mg
- Vitamin D: 0 IU

CONCLUSION

In conclusion, this Osteoporosis Diet Cookbook serves as a comprehensive guide for individuals seeking to manage osteoporosis through dietary choices. By emphasizing nutrient-rich foods, anti-inflammatory ingredients, and delicious recipes, this cookbook provides practical solutions to enhance bone health and overall well-being. From nutritious breakfast options to satisfying dinner recipes and delightful desserts, each dish is carefully crafted to provide essential nutrients like calcium, vitamin D, and protein while minimizing inflammatory factors that can exacerbate osteoporosis.

Adopting and adapting to this diet offers more than just physical benefits; it empowers individuals to take control of their health and improve their quality of life. With dedication and perseverance, incorporating these recipes into daily meals can not only alleviate symptoms of osteoporosis but also foster a positive relationship with food and self-care. Remember, small changes today can lead to significant improvements tomorrow. By nourishing your body with wholesome ingredients and flavorful dishes, you're investing in a healthier, happier future. So, let this cookbook be your companion on the journey to better bone health, and may each recipe inspire you to embrace a lifestyle that prioritizes wellness and vitality.

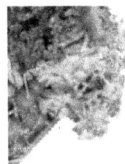

WEEKLY MEAL PLANNER

			GROCERY LIST
MONDAY	BREAKFAST		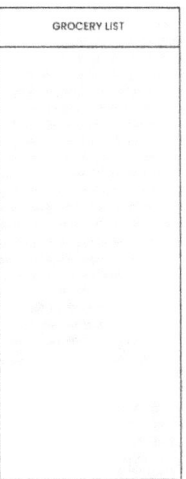
	LUNCH		
	DINNER		
TUESDAY	BREAKFAST		
	LUNCH		
	DINNER		
WEDNESDAY	BREAKFAST		
	LUNCH		
	DINNER		
THURSDAY	BREAKFAST		
	LUNCH		
	DINNER		
FRIDAY	BREAKFAST		SNACKS
	LUNCH		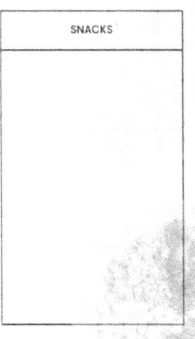
	DINNER		
SARTURDAY	BREAKFAST		
	LUNCH		
	DINNER		
SUNDAY	BREAKFAST		
	LUNCH		
	DINNER		

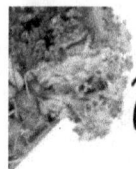

WEEKLY MEAL PLANNER

				GROCERY LIST
MONDAY	BREAKFAST			
	LUNCH			
	DINNER			
TUESDAY	BREAKFAST			
	LUNCH			
	DINNER			
WEDNESDAY	BREAKFAST			
	LUNCH			
	DINNER			
THURSDAY	BREAKFAST			
	LUNCH			
	DINNER			
FRIDAY	BREAKFAST			
	LUNCH			SNACKS
	DINNER			
SARTURDAY	BREAKFAST			
	LUNCH			
	DINNER			
SUNDAY	BREAKFAST			
	LUNCH			
	DINNER			

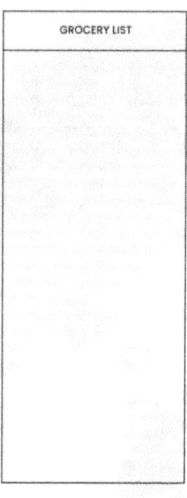

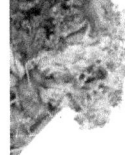

WEEKLY MEAL PLANNER

MONDAY	BREAKFAST	
	LUNCH	
	DINNER	
TUESDAY	BREAKFAST	
	LUNCH	
	DINNER	
WEDNESDAY	BREAKFAST	
	LUNCH	
	DINNER	
THURSDAY	BREAKFAST	
	LUNCH	
	DINNER	
FRIDAY	BREAKFAST	
	LUNCH	
	DINNER	
SARTURDAY	BREAKFAST	
	LUNCH	
	DINNER	
SUNDAY	BREAKFAST	
	LUNCH	
	DINNER	

GROCERY LIST

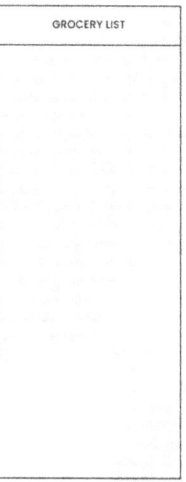

SNACKS

WEEKLY MEAL PLANNER

			GROCERY LIST
MONDAY	BREAKFAST		
	LUNCH		
	DINNER		
TUESDAY	BREAKFAST		
	LUNCH		
	DINNER		
WEDNESDAY	BREAKFAST		
	LUNCH		
	DINNER		
THURSDAY	BREAKFAST		
	LUNCH		
	DINNER		
FRIDAY	BREAKFAST		SNACKS
	LUNCH		
	DINNER		
SARTURDAY	BREAKFAST		
	LUNCH		
	DINNER		
SUNDAY	BREAKFAST		
	LUNCH		
	DINNER		

WEEKLY MEAL PLANNER

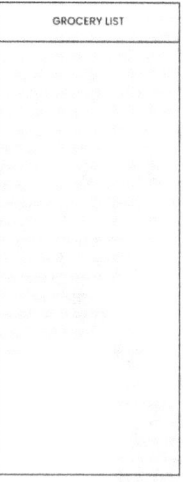

MONDAY	BREAKFAST	
	LUNCH	
	DINNER	
TUESDAY	BREAKFAST	
	LUNCH	
	DINNER	
WEDNESDAY	BREAKFAST	
	LUNCH	
	DINNER	
THURSDAY	BREAKFAST	
	LUNCH	
	DINNER	
FRIDAY	BREAKFAST	
	LUNCH	
	DINNER	
SARTURDAY	BREAKFAST	
	LUNCH	
	DINNER	
SUNDAY	BREAKFAST	
	LUNCH	
	DINNER	

GROCERY LIST

SNACKS

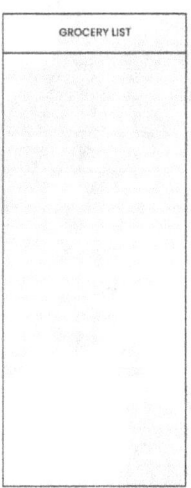

WEEKLY MEAL PLANNER

			GROCERY LIST
MONDAY	BREAKFAST		
	LUNCH		
	DINNER		
TUESDAY	BREAKFAST		
	LUNCH		
	DINNER		
WEDNESDAY	BREAKFAST		
	LUNCH		
	DINNER		
THURSDAY	BREAKFAST		
	LUNCH		
	DINNER		
FRIDAY	BREAKFAST		SNACKS
	LUNCH		
	DINNER		
SARTURDAY	BREAKFAST		
	LUNCH		
	DINNER		
SUNDAY	BREAKFAST		
	LUNCH		
	DINNER		

WEEKLY MEAL PLANNER

				GROCERY LIST
MONDAY	BREAKFAST			
	LUNCH			
	DINNER			
TUESDAY	BREAKFAST			
	LUNCH			
	DINNER			
WEDNESDAY	BREAKFAST			
	LUNCH			
	DINNER			
THURSDAY	BREAKFAST			
	LUNCH			
	DINNER			
FRIDAY	BREAKFAST			
	LUNCH			SNACKS
	DINNER			
SARTURDAY	BREAKFAST			
	LUNCH			
	DINNER			
SUNDAY	BREAKFAST			
	LUNCH			
	DINNER			

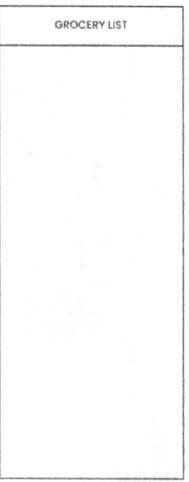

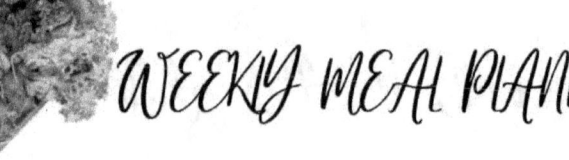

WEEKLY MEAL PLANNER

				GROCERY LIST
MONDAY	BREAKFAST			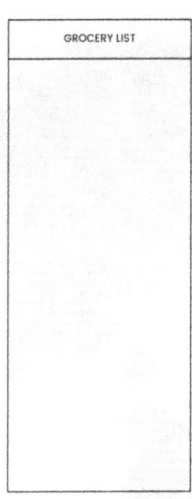
	LUNCH			
	DINNER			
TUESDAY	BREAKFAST			
	LUNCH			
	DINNER			
WEDNESDAY	BREAKFAST			
	LUNCH			
	DINNER			
THURSDAY	BREAKFAST			
	LUNCH			
	DINNER			
FRIDAY	BREAKFAST			SNACKS
	LUNCH			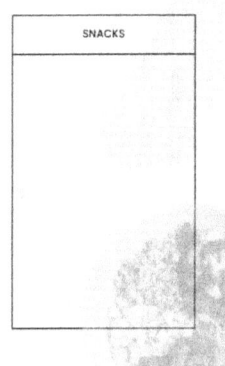
	DINNER			
SARTURDAY	BREAKFAST			
	LUNCH			
	DINNER			
SUNDAY	BREAKFAST			
	LUNCH			
	DINNER			

WEEKLY MEAL PLANNER

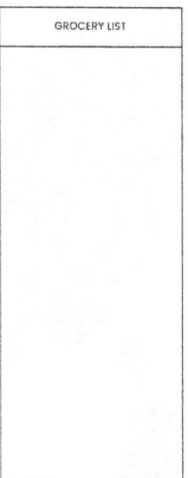

			GROCERY LIST
MONDAY	BREAKFAST		
	LUNCH		
	DINNER		
TUESDAY	BREAKFAST		
	LUNCH		
	DINNER		
WEDNESDAY	BREAKFAST		
	LUNCH		
	DINNER		
THURSDAY	BREAKFAST		
	LUNCH		
	DINNER		
FRIDAY	BREAKFAST		
	LUNCH		SNACKS
	DINNER		
SARTURDAY	BREAKFAST		
	LUNCH		
	DINNER		
SUNDAY	BREAKFAST		
	LUNCH		
	DINNER		

WEEKLY MEAL PLANNER

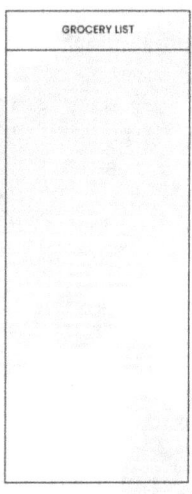

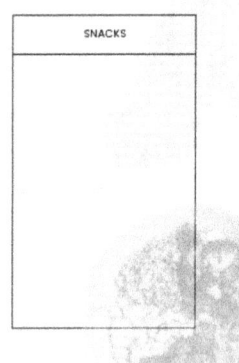

			GROCERY LIST
MONDAY	BREAKFAST		
	LUNCH		
	DINNER		
TUESDAY	BREAKFAST		
	LUNCH		
	DINNER		
WEDNESDAY	BREAKFAST		
	LUNCH		
	DINNER		
THURSDAY	BREAKFAST		
	LUNCH		
	DINNER		
FRIDAY	BREAKFAST		
	LUNCH		SNACKS
	DINNER		
SARTURDAY	BREAKFAST		
	LUNCH		
	DINNER		
SUNDAY	BREAKFAST		
	LUNCH		
	DINNER		

WEEKLY MEAL PLANNER

MONDAY	BREAKFAST	
	LUNCH	
	DINNER	
TUESDAY	BREAKFAST	
	LUNCH	
	DINNER	
WEDNESDAY	BREAKFAST	
	LUNCH	
	DINNER	
THURSDAY	BREAKFAST	
	LUNCH	
	DINNER	
FRIDAY	BREAKFAST	
	LUNCH	
	DINNER	
SARTURDAY	BREAKFAST	
	LUNCH	
	DINNER	
SUNDAY	BREAKFAST	
	LUNCH	
	DINNER	

GROCERY LIST

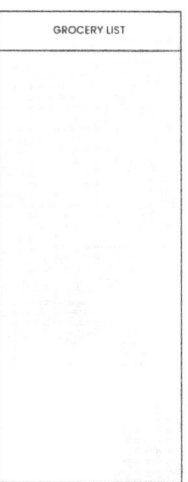

SNACKS

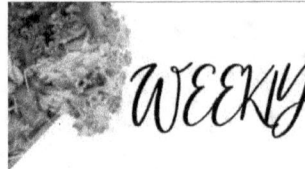

WEEKLY MEAL PLANNER

			GROCERY LIST
MONDAY	BREAKFAST		
	LUNCH		
	DINNER		
TUESDAY	BREAKFAST		
	LUNCH		
	DINNER		
WEDNESDAY	BREAKFAST		
	LUNCH		
	DINNER		
THURSDAY	BREAKFAST		
	LUNCH		
	DINNER		
FRIDAY	BREAKFAST		SNACKS
	LUNCH		
	DINNER		
SARTURDAY	BREAKFAST		
	LUNCH		
	DINNER		
SUNDAY	BREAKFAST		
	LUNCH		
	DINNER		

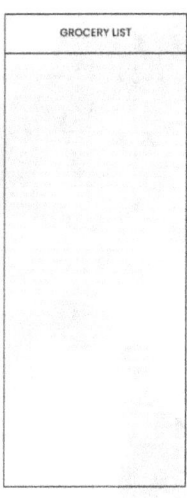

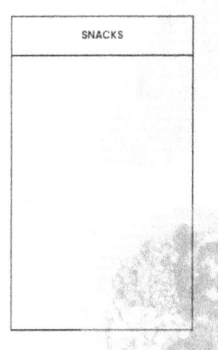

WEEKLY MEAL PLANNER

MONDAY	BREAKFAST	
	LUNCH	
	DINNER	
TUESDAY	BREAKFAST	
	LUNCH	
	DINNER	
WEDNESDAY	BREAKFAST	
	LUNCH	
	DINNER	
THURSDAY	BREAKFAST	
	LUNCH	
	DINNER	
FRIDAY	BREAKFAST	
	LUNCH	
	DINNER	
SARTURDAY	BREAKFAST	
	LUNCH	
	DINNER	
SUNDAY	BREAKFAST	
	LUNCH	
	DINNER	

GROCERY LIST

SNACKS

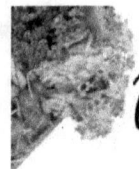

WEEKLY MEAL PLANNER

			GROCERY LIST
MONDAY	BREAKFAST		
	LUNCH		
	DINNER		
TUESDAY	BREAKFAST		
	LUNCH		
	DINNER		
WEDNESDAY	BREAKFAST		
	LUNCH		
	DINNER		
THURSDAY	BREAKFAST		
	LUNCH		
	DINNER		
FRIDAY	BREAKFAST		
	LUNCH		SNACKS
	DINNER		
SARTURDAY	BREAKFAST		
	LUNCH		
	DINNER		
SUNDAY	BREAKFAST		
	LUNCH		
	DINNER		

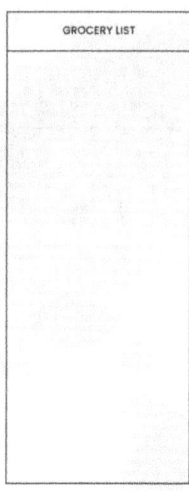

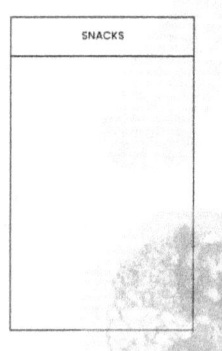

.